Starting Your Personal Fitness Program

Ann Ward, Ph.D.
Assistant Professor of Medicine

James M. Rippe, M.D.
Assistant Professor of Medicine

**Division of Cardiovascular Medicine
and Exercise Physiology Laboratory
University of Massachusetts Medical Center
Worcester, Massachusetts**

J. B. Lippincott Company   Philadelphia
London   Mexico City   New York
St. Louis   São Paulo   Sydney

The Health–Fitness Link

In this booklet we will explain why regular exercise is important, give you guidelines for starting your personal fitness program, and present ideas on how you can keep going and enjoy the benefits of a fitness program.

People exercise for many different reasons, including the desire to stay in shape, to control their weight, and to feel and look better. But most people exercise to improve their health. In our mechanized society work and home activities do not provide enough of the type of exercise that is beneficial for cardiovascular health. Regular exercise contributes to overall good health in many ways. The health benefits include reduction in the risk of heart attack, weight control, slowing of bone loss (osteoporosis), decreased stress and anxiety, and improved sense of well-being. In addition, exercise increases stamina and resistance to fatigue and tones muscles. There is recent evidence that exercise may help to reduce cancer risk. Some of the many health benefits of exercise are listed in Table 1.

TABLE 1. Benefits of Exercise

Improves aerobic capacity	May slow bone loss (osteoporosis)
May lower blood pressure	Improves self-image
May lower cholesterol	Helps to decrease anxiety and depression
Burns calories to help in weight control	Improves sense of well-being
May help control appetite	

Still, exercise is only one component of a total fitness program. A truly comprehensive program should also include attention to risk factors for heart disease such as high blood pressure, high cholesterol, and cigarette smoking; proper nutrition; weight control; musculoskeletal strength; flexibility; and lifestyle habits. This booklet is designed to provide information regarding the link between health and fitness and to provide guidelines for a safe, appropriate total fitness program.

Getting Started

Many individuals who would like to start an exercise program do not know how to begin. A total fitness program requires planning to ensure maximum safety, prevent injuries, and gain optimal benefits. This section of this booklet focuses on developing a plan for starting an exercise program, the kinds of tests to obtain prior to starting exercise, the type and amount of exercise, and how to purchase proper equipment.

Initiating a personal fitness program can be looked upon as a series of five steps. These are

STEP I: Pre-program evaluation
STEP II: Develop a plan
STEP III: Test your fitness level
STEP IV: Choose the right exercise
STEP V: Exercise prescription

Pre-Program Evaluation

Your physician has probably discussed with you the importance of exercise and the need to develop a safe program. In determining the safety of exercise for you, it is important to consider your individual and family history for heart disease. This includes information on risk factors such as high blood pressure, elevated cholesterol, cigarette smoking, and obesity. Your physician may also have recommended an exercise stress test before you begin your fitness program. The exercise stress test is one of the best ways to make sure that an exercise program is safe for you. This test involves walking or running on a treadmill while a physician watches your electrocardiogram (ECG). The guidelines published by the American College of Sports Medicine recommend that previously inactive individuals over age 45 should have this test before starting a new exercise program. If you are younger and have been very inactive or have risk factors for heart disease, undergoing the test is a good idea. Of course, there are some exceptions, and your physician should make the final decision.

Developing a Plan

When your physician has approved you for exercise and you have decided to start a program, you should develop a plan that will help you optimize benefits and avoid injuries and discouragement.

First, you should choose an activity that you enjoy and in which you have some skill and ability. The activity should also be convenient to participate in. If you must travel a long distance or if you have trouble finding partners, you will be less likely to continue the program. Individual sports such as jogging, walking, and stationary cycling, which do not require special facilities and other players, are obviously more convenient.

Another important factor in beginning an exercise program is finding a convenient, regular time to exercise. Some people find that mornings are the best time to exercise, before they get involved in other daily activities. Others like to take an exercise break at lunchtime or during the evening after work. Following a regular schedule helps to make exercise a habit.

After selecting an activity and a convenient time for exercise, you need to determine exactly how much and how hard you should exercise in order to achieve benefits. This is called an exercise prescription and is based on your current health, physical capability, and goals. The guidelines in this booklet along with recommendations from your physician can help you develop a safe, effective program.

Should you join an exercise facility or club? This is largely a matter of personal style and preference. We have found that people are more likely to continue in exercise programs if they exercise with others rather than alone, so we generally recommend that people find friends to exercise with. Exercise clubs and facilities provide group activities and professionals who can guide you in your exercise program. Before joining a club, you should consider the convenience of the location, the hours that the facility is open, and how crowded the facility is during the hours you want to exercise. It is a good idea to have a trial exercise session or class at the time you would regularly participate to determine the availability of space, equipment, and locker facilities. Also, ask about certification and training of staff.

Once you start a fitness program, it is a good idea to keep an exercise log such as the one on the inside back cover of this booklet. Record your daily activity along with subjective impressions about how you felt during the session and any problems you encountered. The exercise log also is a good method for charting your progress.

Remember that it may have taken years for you to get out of shape. Take your time and progress slowly to avoid injury and discouragement while you get back in shape.

Testing Your Fitness Level

Knowledge of your physical fitness level before you begin your exercise program can help you start at an appropriate level and set reasonable goals. Your fitness level also provides a baseline against which you can compare subsequent tests as you progress. If you belong to an exercise facility or club, a staff member should be able to administer some simple tests to estimate your fitness. Based on your performance on these tests, an exercise specialist can design an exercise program (called an exercise prescription) for you. We will present the Rockport Fitness Walking

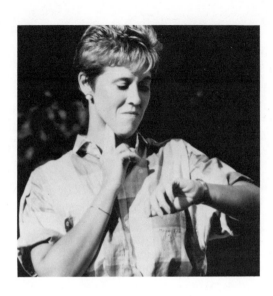

Fig. 1 Taking the carotid pulse

Test* for estimating your cardiovascular fitness level. Later in this booklet we will describe how the results of this test can be used to develop your exercise program.

The Rockport Fitness Walking Test

The Rockport Fitness Walking Test provides an accurate assessment of aerobic capacity. This test was developed at the Exercise Physiology Laboratory and Department of Exercise Science at the University of Massachusetts. It offers a safe way to test aerobic capacity using the most common form of exercise—walking. The test can be used with any age group and at any level of fitness and does not require expensive equipment.

To take the Rockport Fitness Walking Test, you first need to know how to count your pulse or heart rate. Knowing how to take your pulse will also be useful in monitoring your exercise program.

To take your heart rate, feel the pulse of the artery at your wrist (radial pulse) or throat (carotid pulse). The radial pulse can be found by placing two fingers over the radial artery just inside your wrist on the thumb side of your arm. The carotid pulse can be found by inserting your fingers softly into your neck at either side of your Adam's apple just below your jaw. When you have found your pulse, time it with your watch. Count the number of beats for 15 seconds, then multiply by 4 to derive the number of heartbeats per minute. (For example, if while relaxing you count 18 beats in 15 seconds, your resting heart rate is 18 × 4 or 72 beats per minute.) Practice taking your pulse a few times because it is an important part of the test and your subsequent exercise program.

The Rockport Fitness Walking Test procedures involve the following steps:

1. Locate a measured track or measure out 1 mile at any convenient, level location. You will need a watch capable of recording time in minutes and seconds.
2. Stretch and warmup for 5 to 10 minutes. Stretching information is provided later in this booklet. You should wear shoes and clothing that are comfortable for walking.
3. Walk 1 mile as fast as possible. Maintain a steady pace. Time your walk with your watch to the nearest second.
4. Take a 15-second heart rate count immediately upon completing the mile. The 15-second count is multiplied by 4 to obtain the heart rate in beats per minute. Record your results as follows:
   Age: _____ years
   Time to walk 1 mile: _____ minutes, _____ seconds

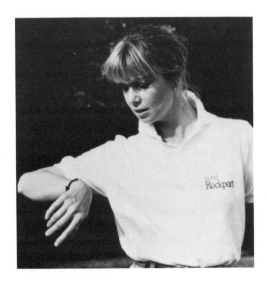

Fig. 2 Record your time at the end of the mile.

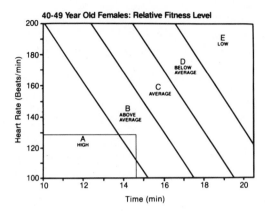

Fig. 3 Fitness level sample

Heart rate at end of mile: _____ beats/minute
(Remember, count your pulse for 15 seconds, then multiply by 4 to
determine your heart rate for 1 minute.)

5. To find your fitness level, locate the appropriate age and sex chart
from the Relative Fitness Level charts at the end of this booklet
and draw a vertical line from your mile time to intersect with a
horizontal line from your heart rate. This point of intersection
identifies your relative fitness level.

For example, a 45-year-old woman had a one-mile walk time
of 14 minutes, 30 seconds, and her heart rate at the end of the mile
was 128 beats per minute. She fell into the "B" or *above average*
category (see Figure 3).

Choosing the Right Exercise

There are basically two types of exercise: aerobic and anaerobic. Under-
standing what these are will help you select the right combination of
activities to achieve your goals and optimize cardiovascular and health
benefits.

1. *Aerobic exercise.* Aerobic means "in the presence of air." The
major source of energy production and the most efficient system
the body has for endurance exercise is the aerobic system, which
requires oxygen. Aerobic activities are those that require use of
large muscle groups, are rhythmic in nature, and can be maintained for 20 to 30 minutes. These are the exercises most beneficial
for your heart and for weight control. Examples of aerobic exer-

cises include jogging, fitness walking, cycling, rope jumping, aerobic dancing, swimming, cross-country skiing, and rowing.

2. *Anaerobic exercise.* Anaerobic means "without oxygen." When you perform short bursts of intense activity, most of the energy is produced without a supply of oxygen. This process is fast but inefficient and cannot be maintained for very long. These activities do not burn many Calories and thus are not effective for weight loss. These activities also do not benefit your heart since they are not sustained. They may, however, help develop muscular strength, skill, speed, and agility. Examples of anaerobic exercises include sprinting and weight lifting.

Sports and recreational activities such as softball, tennis, and basketball are frequently a combination of aerobic and anaerobic exercise. These are activities in which skill is important. They provide pleasure and enjoyment, but are not sustained enough to provide the most cardiovascular benefit.

Both aerobic and anaerobic activities are important for total fitness. However, aerobic activities should make up the core of your fitness program because these activities promote cardiovascular health benefits and weight control. Supplement your aerobic activity with other forms of exercise to increase muscle strength, flexibility, skill, and enjoyment.

When you have decided what types of activities you will participate in, it is important to get proper equipment. If you decide to jog, for example, the most important purchase is a good pair of running shoes. You should anticipate spending $40 to $70 for these. For fitness walking, the only essential purchase is a pair of shoes designed specifically for this activity. For outside exercise in cold or rainy weather, some type of foul-weather gear is essential. A nylon running suit will substantially reduce windchill and some of the newer water-resistant fabrics will keep you dry. Check with friends who successfully participate in the type of exercise you have chosen or with athletic stores to learn which equipment is recommended.

Exercise Prescription

Now that you have decided which types of activities you will participate in, you need to know how hard, how often, and how long you should exercise during the aerobic or training phase. We refer to this as an *exercise prescription,* which is as important to follow as a prescription for

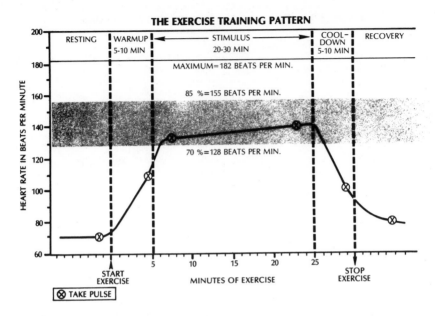

Fig. 4 The exercise training pattern (From Zohman LR: Beyond Diet: Exercise Your Way to Fitness and Heart Health. CPC International, Englewood Cliffs, NJ, 1979.)

medicine in terms of improving your cardiovascular endurance and avoiding injuries.

An exercise session should consist of three phases. These are the warmup, the training period, and the cooldown (Figure 4). The warmup and cooldown should include stretching and low intensity exercise. The training period may involve aerobic activities, games and recreational activities, or muscular-strength training.

Intensity. Intensity refers to how hard you work during the training phase. Heart rate provides the best way to monitor your exercise intensity or level of exertion. The activity should be at an intensity that raises your heart rate to 60 to 85% of your predicted maximum heart rate. This is called your *target heart rate zone*. If you have been inactive, you should start your new exercise program at 60% of your maximum heart rate. As you adjust to your new program, you should gradually increase your intensity to 70 to 85%. You should already know how to take your pulse if you took the Rockport Fitness Walking Test. Use the following steps to calculate your target heart rate zone:

TABLE 2. Target Heart Rate Zone (Beats/min)

Age (yrs)	Target zone (beats/min)			Average max HR (100%)
	60%	70%	80%	
20	120	140	170	200
25	117	137	166	195
30	114	133	162	190
35	111	130	157	185
40	108	126	153	180
45	105	123	149	175
50	102	119	145	170
55	99	116	140	165
60	96	112	136	160
65	93	109	132	155
70	90	105	128	150

1. Compute your maximum predicted heart rate. The easiest way to do this is to take 220 beats per minute and subtract your age. (For example, if you are 45 years old, your predicted maximum heart rate is 220 minus 45, or 175 beats per minute.)
2. Determine your target heart rate zone. This involves multiplying your predicted maximum heart rate by 60 to 85%. (For the 45 year old, the target zone lies between 175 × .60 (60%) and 175 × .85 (85%), or between 105 and 149 beats per minute.)

Table 2 will help you determine your target heart rate zone. These heart rates are estimates and should be used as general guidelines. You should also monitor how you feel. If you are breathless while you exercise or still exhausted two hours after you complete your exercise, you are working too hard and should decrease your intensity.

We recommend that you take your pulse for 15 seconds every 5 minutes when you begin an exercise program. You should start counting your pulse immediately upon stopping your exercise to get an accurate estimate of your intensity. If you are below your target heart rate, you should exercise harder (for example, increase your walking or jogging pace), and if you are above your target, you should exercise easier or decrease your intensity (for example, decrease your walking or jogging pace). Eventually you will be able to accurately estimate your heart rate with fewer actual measurements.

As your fitness level increases, you will find that you must exercise harder to keep your heart rate in the target zone. This is because your heart and muscles have become more efficient and are better able to handle the intensity of the exercise.

Most medications will have no effect on exercise. However, if you have specific questions, you should speak to your doctor. One commonly prescribed class of medications does influence how your heart responds to exercise. These medicines fall in the general class of drugs called *beta blockers*, which are often prescribed for angina (chest pain associated with heart disease) and high blood pressure. These medications may make it difficult to reach your target heart rate zone. If you are taking a beta blocker, your physician can help you adjust your exercise program.

Frequency. Frequency is the number of times you exercise per week. To be effective, aerobic exercise should be performed at least 3 times per week. Sessions should be spread evenly throughout the week to allow your body to recover. For example, if you are exercising 3 days per week you should allow a day of rest between your sessions. Exercising 6 to 7 times a week may induce more improvement than 3 days per week, but may also increase your chance of injury. Low-impact or low-intensity exercise such as walking or stationary cycling can be performed 5 to 6 times per week with minimal risk of injury.

Duration. Duration is the length of time you exercise at your target heart rate zone. The duration of exercise should start out at 10 to 15 minutes for beginners and progress to 20 to 60 minutes of continuous activity. The duration of exercise sessions will depend on your goals and the intensity of exercise. If your goal is to lose weight, you should exercise at the lower end of your target heart rate zone for a longer duration in order to burn more calories.

To summarize, for the aerobic part of your exercise program you should gradually build up to 20 to 60 minutes of exercise at 60 to 85% of your maximum heart rate for 3 to 5 days per week. This amount of exercise will provide an optimal level of fitness. Your exact exercise prescription will be based on your goals and available time.

TABLE 3. Exercise Prescription Guidelines

Frequency	3–5 days per week
Intensity	60–85% maximum heart rate
Duration	20–60 minutes per session
Mode	Aerobic activities, including walking, jogging, swimming, cycling, and so forth

Warmup, Cooldown, and Flexibility

Warmup. Warming up before your workout and cooling down after it are very important aspects of total fitness. A proper warmup period allows your heart to gradually accelerate into the training zone. Stretching and flexibility exercises should be included to develop and maintain adequate range of motion in all joints of the body. The warmup should also include low-intensity exercise, such as walking, designed to gradually prepare the muscles for higher-intensity exercise. Failure to stretch and warmup may lead to a variety of problems ranging from minor inconveniences such as stiffness to major problems such as musculoskeletal injuries or dangerous heart rhythms.

What constitutes a proper warmup? At least 5 to 10 minutes of gradually progressive exertion. The best form of exertion for warmup is the exercise you are about to perform, but at a lower intensity. For example, if your workout is running, gradually warm up through progressively more vigorous walking and jogging. If you are about to play tennis, warm up with jogging and some light ground strokes and volleying.

Cooldown. Proper cooling down is just as important as warming up. The principles are very similar except that in this situation your goal is a gradual deceleration of your heart rate rather than acceleration. The proper cooling down should take 5 to 10 minutes and is followed by post-exercise stretches. The cooling-down period helps to keep the blood flowing back to the heart and decreases the likelihood of lightheadedness and abnormal heart rhythms. Cooling down also helps prevent stiffness and is essential to help the muscles clear waste products.

Flexibility. Stretching exercises are important for developing and maintaining adequate range of motion in the joints of the body. Some experts believe that stretching before exercising may help prevent injury. Stretching exercises should be performed both before and after exercise to enhance flexibility. They are generally performed at the beginning of the warmup and at the end of the cooldown. A few considerations will help you derive the most benefit from your stretching.

1. Select stretches that are specific for the exercise you are about to undertake. Analyze the muscle groups used in the sport or activity you are about to perform and stretch these muscle groups. For example, walking and running use the large muscle groups of the front and back of the leg (quadriceps and hamstring muscles) as

well as those of the lower back. Stretches should focus on these muscles. Other activities such as swimming and rowing involve more muscle groups. It is also important to stretch before participating in sports activities such as tennis and golf.

2. Perform stretches correctly. Stretching exercises should be performed slowly with gradual progression to greater ranges of motion. A slow movement into the stretch position should be followed with a static stretch that is sustained for 20 to 30 seconds. You should never stretch to the point of actual pain, and if at any point you experience pain, you should ease away from the stretch. A wide variety of illustrated stretching programs are available in fitness books. One that we frequently recommend is entitled *Stretching* by Bob Anderson and is available in most bookstores.

3. Breathe in and out regularly as you perform the stretches and avoid holding your breath. Focusing on your breathing can also help you relax and get the most out of your stretch.

Aerobic Conditioning

Aerobic conditioning is the cornerstone of a comprehensive fitness program. The most common aerobic sports include fitness walking, jogging or running, cycling or stationary cycling, swimming, rowing, rope jumping, aerobic dance, and cross-country skiing. All of these activities are excellent for your heart and muscles. The choice boils down to personal preference, availability of facilities and equipment, and season of the year.

TABLE 4.   16-Week Walking Program

Week	Pace (min/mile [mph])	Distance (miles)	Time (min:sec)	Heart Rate (% of max)	Frequency (days/wk)
1	24:00 [2.5]	.75	18:00	60	5–6
2	24:00 [2.5]	1	24:00	60	5–6
3–4	20:00 [3.0]	1.25	25:00	60–70	5–6
5–6	20:00 [3.0]	1.5	30:00	60–70	5–6
7–8	20:00 [3.0]	2	40:00	60–70	5–6
9–10	18:30 [3.25]	2	37:00	70	5–6
11–12	18:30 [3.25]	2.25	41:38	70	5–6
13–14	18:30 [3.25]	2.5	46:15	70	5–6
15–16	17:00 [3.5]	2.5	42:30	70–80	5–6

TABLE 5. 20-Week Walking Program

Week	Pace (min/mile [mph])	Distance (miles)	Time (min:sec)	Heart Rate (% of max)	Frequency (days/wk)
1–2	18:30 [3.25]	2	37:00	60–70	4–6
3–4	18:30 [3.25]	2.5	46:15	60–70	4–6
5–6	17:00 [3.5]	2.5	42:30	70	4–6
7–8	17:00 [3.5]	2.75	46:45	70	4–6
9–12	16:00 [3.75]	2.75	44:00	70–80	4–6
13–16	16:00 [3.75]	3	48:00	70–80	4–6
17–20	15:00 [4.0]	3	45:00	80	4–6

Walking. Walking is an excellent and very underrated form of aerobic exercise. We have found in our laboratory that even young, fit persons can attain their target heart rate by fitness walking. If you are over 40 years old and have been inactive, we recommend that you start with a walking program. The programs outlined below are designed to get you started. The 16-week starter program is designed for individuals scoring "E" or *low* and "D" or *below average* on the Rockport Fitness Walking Test. The 20-week program is designed for individuals scoring "C" (*average*) or "B" or "A" (*above average* or *high*) on the Rockport Fitness Walking Test. The paces listed in these tables are only approximations. Your walking pace should be determined by the speed that keeps your heart rate in the target zone.

Jogging. Jogging or running are excellent aerobic-conditioning activities. The sample jogging program in Table 6 is designed for individuals who fall at least in the "C" or *average* category on the Relative Fitness Level

TABLE 6. 20-Week Jogging Program

Week	Walk/Jog (min)	Intervals (#)	Time (min)	Heart Rate (% of max)	Frequency (days/wk)
1–2	2/1	8	24	60–70	3–4
3–4	2/2	6	24	70	3–4
5–6	1/2	8	24	70	3–4
7–8	1/3	6	24	70–80	3–4
9–10	1/3	7	28	70–80	3–4
11–12	1/4	6	30	70–80	3–4
13–14	1/5	5	30	70–80	3–4
15–16	1/7	4	32	80	3–4
17–18	1/9	3	30	80	3–4
19–20	1/10	3	33	80	3–4

chart. Choose a jogging pace that is comfortable and gets your heart rate in the target zone. A rule of thumb for pacing yourself is that you should be able to carry on a conversation with a companion. Start out with a walk/jog interval program and gradually increase the duration of the jogging intervals until you can jog the total distance. Check your heart rate immediately after the jogging intervals to determine if you are exercising at the correct intensity.

Cycling. Cycling is also an excellent way to achieve aerobic conditioning. Stationary cycling is a good way to maintain your conditioning during the winter months and is beneficial for individuals with knee and back problems. Many good stationary cycles are available commercially. You should choose one that has a weighted flywheel that allows you to adjust the resistance. For stationary cycling the resistance should be set at a level that raises your heart rate to the target zone. The pedal rate typically ranges from 50 to 80 revolutions per minute (RPM).

TABLE 7. 20-Week Stationary Cycling Program

Week	Heart Rate (% of max)	Time (min)	Frequency (days/wk)
1–2	60	18	3
3–4	60	20	3
5–6	60–70	22	3
7–8	60–70	24	3
9–10	60–70	26	3
11–12	70–80	28	3
13–14	70–80	30	3
15–16	70–80	32	3
17–18	80	34	3
19–20	80	36	3

(Adapted with permission from Rippe JM, Southmayd W: The Sports Performance Factors. New York, GP Putnam and Sons, 1986.)

Swimming. Swimming is one of the most popular sports activities in this country. It has been called the perfect total-body aerobic exercise because you use upper body muscles as well as lower body muscles. In addition to the advantages offered by all forms of aerobic exercise, swimming has an advantage of its own. Because of the cushioning effect of water, there is less stress on bones, joints, and muscles than with other activities. Thus swimming is a very good activity for the elderly and those with joint problems. Also, many swimmers profess that swimming is re-

TABLE 8. 20-Week Swimming Program

Week	Distance (yards)	Heart Rate (% of max)	Frequency (days/wk)
1–2	150	60–65	3
3–4	200	60–65	3
5–6	250	65–70	3
7–8	300	65–70	3
9–10	400	70–75	3
11–12	500	70–75	3
13–14	600	70–75	3
15–16	750	75–80	3
17–18	900	75–80	3
19–20	1000	75–80	3

(Adapted with permission from Rippe JM, Southmayd W: The Sports Performance Factors. New York, GP Putnam and Sons, 1986.)

laxing. Getting to a facility with a swimming pool, however, is frequently inconvenient.

A 20-week swimming program is presented in Table 8. Use different strokes to add variety and rest periods to your workout. The progression is only a suggestion. Some people may want to build up distance more slowly.

Rowing. Rowing and stationary rowing are becoming increasingly popular. Like swimming, rowing is a non-impact exercise and consequently has a low risk of injury. An advantage of rowing is that it uses leg, arm, back, and abdominal muscles in each stroke. Rowing is an excellent cardiovascular fitness activity used alone. It can also be used as a supplement to weight-bearing activities. Similar guidelines for frequency, intensity, and duration should be followed. Resistance can be adjusted in some rowing machines. Adjust resistance and stroke rate to achieve your target heart rate zone.

Cross-Country Skiing. Cross-country skiing is a seasonal activity. Skiing adds variety and enjoyment when used in conjunction with other forms of aerobic exercise. You can use your usual training heart rate zone as a guide. You may want to pause periodically to rest and enjoy the environment. Remember to drink fluids regularly while skiing because breathing cold dry air can lead to dehydration.

Environmental Considerations

When engaging in outdoor activities you should take appropriate precautions for special weather conditions. The heat load increases with temperature, humidity, direct sunlight, and your level of exertion. Wind aids in cooling through evaporation of sweat. On hot, humid days you should follow these recommendations to avoid heat stress:

1. Wear light-colored, light-weight, loose-fitting clothing to improve sweat evaporation and heat loss.
2. Exercise during the cooler parts of the day such as early morning or during the evening after the sun has gone down.
3. Decrease intensity or duration of exercise. Exercise heart rate is higher in hot conditions and provides a good monitor of the heat load. Decrease your pace to keep your exercise heart rate in its normal range. Monitor your heart rate more frequently.
4. Drink plenty of water before, during, and after exercise. Most people do not need extra salt because the normal diet provides an adequate amount of salt intake.
5. Do not wear rubber or plastic suits, sweatshirts, or sweatpants. This clothing will not help you lose weight any faster by making you sweat more; the weight you lose will be quickly replaced as you begin drinking fluids again. Moreover this type of clothing can cause dangerously high body temperatures, possibly resulting in heat stroke.

Cold weather presents different problems than hot weather. Wind increases the cooling effect of temperature. This cooling is called the *windchill* effect. Use the following guidelines to avoid problems and make exercising on cold days more enjoyable. Cardiac patients and older individuals should exercise indoors when the windchill temperature is below 20 degrees Fahrenheit.

1. Wear clothing that protects the head and extremities as well as the rest of the body.
2. Do not overdress, but wear layers of clothing that can be unzipped or removed as you get warmer.
3. On windy days start out against the wind and return with the wind. A nylon running suit will help reduce the windchill.
4. Try to stay dry. Water increases the rate of heat loss. Remove damp or wet clothing as soon as possible.

Musculoskeletal Strength Training

Although aerobic exercise is more beneficial to the heart than other types of exercise, improving strength and muscular endurance is also a very important part of a well-rounded exercise program. As an addition to aerobic conditioning, strength programs can make your training more enjoyable, improve your appearance by toning muscles, improve your total fitness, improve your performance in recreational and leisure time sports, and help prevent injuries.

There are three basic types of muscular strength and power building regimens: isometric, isotonic, and isokinetic.

Isometric exercise involves contracting the muscle in one position against an immovable resistance. An example of this is pushing against a wall as hard as you can. Isometric training is discouraged because these regimens can cause dangerous elevations in blood pressure while the contraction is being held, and they do not really enhance athletic performance.

In isotonic exercise, the muscle contracts through its full range of motion to overcome a fixed resistance. The classic example of isotonic exercise is lifting free weights. Isotonic programs are excellent for building strength and power, but have one major limitation: at different angles the muscles are able to lift different amounts of weight, and so you are limited to lifting the amount of weight that can be hoisted through the weakest part of the range of motion of the particular muscle being exercised.

Variable-resistance isotonic machines have been developed to overcome this problem. Furthermore, using these machines strengthens the muscle when it shortens as well as when it lengthens.

Isokinetic equipment has a variable resistance against a fixed rate of contraction. The muscle is maximally loaded throughout the range of motion.

Strength Training Guidelines

Like aerobic exercise, strength training should be performed 3 days per week on alternate days for 15 to 60 minutes each time. Strength training may be performed as part of an aerobic exercise session or on separate days. Your specific strength-training program will be based on your needs and goals, available equipment, and time. If you have high blood pressure or coronary heart disease or questions about the safety of muscle training for you, consult your physician.

INSTRUCTION: If you are beginning a strength-training program, we strongly recommend that you get instruction from a qualified fitness specialist at an exercise facility. These individuals can instruct you on choosing a strength-training system, learning the proper technique, getting started, and progressing. Proper instruction will optimize your benefits from strength training and minimize your risk of injury.

WARMUP: Stretch for 5 to 10 minutes before each weight-training session. Be sure to stretch each muscle group you plan to exercise during the workout.

FREQUENCY: Strength training should be performed 2 to 3 times per week for any particular muscle group. It can be performed along with your aerobic workout or on alternate days. Allow 48 hours between strength-training workouts to give muscles time to recover.

INTENSITY: Intensity refers to the amount of weight being lifted and the number of repetitions (reps). An exercise specialist should help you choose a proper starting weight. The number of repetitions is based on your goals. We generally recommend a program that emphasizes strength and endurance. For most people this means selecting a weight that can be lifted 8 to 12 times.

DURATION: Duration refers to the number of sets you perform. One set is 8 to 12 repetitions without resting. The number of sets you perform depends on the type of equipment you use and your goals. We normally recommend one to three sets.

PROGRESSIVE OVERLOAD: For a muscle to increase in size and strength, it must be overloaded or exercised at a resistance greater than normal use. As you get stronger, the initial weight will no longer overload the muscle sufficiently. You must increase either your number of repetitions or your weight load to continue overloading the muscle.

SPECIFICITY: Muscular strength and endurance is gained in the muscle groups that are overloaded. The specific muscle groups you exercise should be based on your goals and needs. We recommend a balanced program that exercises both the upper and lower body.

The following rules will help you minimize the risk of injury.

1. Seek instruction to learn proper technique and to develop an appropriate program.

2. Warmup and cool down with stretching. Remember to stretch the muscle groups you will be exercising.
3. Breathe regularly throughout each repetition. The basic rhythm is to inhale with exertion and exhale when returning the weight to the starting position.
4. Use proper mechanics. Use weights that allow you to completely control the movement so that you do not use extraneous body parts to lift the weight.
5. Use consistent rhythm during the set and do not pause between repetitions.
6. *Progress slowly!*

Nutrition and Weight Control

Proper nutrition is an important element of a total health and fitness program. Food provides nourishment and fuel for movement. We know that attention to the foods we eat can play an important role in daily and lifelong performance and health.

What Is the Best Diet?

The American Heart Association has proposed the dietary guidelines in Table 9 for achieving an optimal diet for healthy adults. Because individual nutrient intake varies according to body size, physical activity, metabolic efficiency, and net energy balance, the dietary guidelines are ex-

TABLE 9. American Heart Association Dietary Guidelines

1. *Saturated fat* intake should be less than 10% of Calories.
2. *Total fat* intake should be less than 30% of Calories.
3. *Cholesterol* intake should be less than 100 mg per 1000 Calories, but not to exceed 300 mg per day.
4. *Protein* intake should be approximately 15% of Calories.
5. *Carbohydrate* intake should make up 50–55% or more of Calories with emphasis on increasing sources of complex carbohydrates.
6. *Sodium* intake should be reduced to approximately 1 gram per 1000 Calories, not to exceed 3 grams per day.
7. If alcoholic beverages are consumed, the limit should be 15% of total Calories, not to exceed 1 ounce of alcohol (approximately 2 drinks, beers, or glasses of wine) per day.
8. Total Calories should be sufficient to maintain your best weight.
9. A wide variety of foods should be consumed.

pressed in relationship to caloric intake. For more details, *The American Heart Association Cookbook* (available in most bookstores) provides practical suggestions for implementing these guidelines.

What Is Desirable Body Weight?

Desirable body weight refers to the weight that represents an optimal balance between lean and fat weight. Fat weight should not exceed 20% and 30% of total body weight for men and women, respectively. There are several ways to determine your desirable weight. The most accurate method is underwater weighing, but this is used primarily in laboratories for research purposes. The skinfold technique, although not as accurate as underwater weighing, provides a good estimate of your body fat (Fig. 5). Many exercise facilities have staff who are trained in the skinfold technique. A good estimate of your desirable body weight can be made based on your skinfold fat measurements.

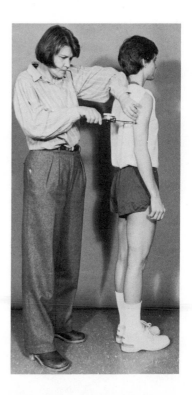

Fig. 5 Taking a skinfold measurement

Another method of estimating your desirable weight involves simple arithmetic as outlined below. The disadvantage of this method is that it fails to account for ranges in muscle mass and frame size.

For men:

1. Record the number of inches in your height over 5 feet and multiply this by 6.
2. Add 106.
   Example: If you are 5'8" tall,
   $8 \times 6 = 48 + 106 = 154$ lbs is your ideal weight.

For women:

1. Record the number of inches in your height over 5 feet and multiply this number by 5.
2. Add 100.
   Example: If you are 5'4" tall,
   $4 \times 5 = 20 + 100 = 120$ lbs is your ideal weight.

How Can You Reach Your Desirable Body Weight?

Until recently, people believed that the major cause of obesity was simply overeating. However, we now know that it is much more complicated. Many factors may predispose a person to weight gain, including genetic, physiological, environmental, and psychosocial influences. Lack of physical activity is also an important factor in weight gain.

The number of Calories consumed compared with the number of Calories expended is referred to as the *energy balance equation*. In order for your weight to remain constant, you must burn the same number of Calories as you take in. If you are gaining weight, you are taking in more Calories than you are burning. These Calories are stored in the body as excess fat.

To lose fat or weight, you must unbalance the energy equation toward greater Calorie expenditure compared with caloric intake. You can accomplish this in the following three ways:

1. Diet: Reduce daily caloric intake below energy expenditure.
2. Exercise: Increase energy expenditure over caloric intake.
3. Combination of diet and exercise.

We have found that the combination of diet and exercise is the ideal weight-loss program. You can lose weight simply by decreasing the amount of food you eat, but, in this situation, you will lose muscle tissue as well as fat. If you drift back to your old eating habits, it is much easier to regain the fat than to rebuild the muscle tissue.

Exercise combined with diet minimizes the loss of muscle tissue associated with dieting so that most of the weight loss is in the form of fat. Exercise also burns Calories, improves appetite control, and promotes a feeling of well-being. Also, recent scientific studies have shown that individuals who combine exercise with diet are more successful in maintaining weight loss.

Weight loss should be consistent and gradual. We generally recommend losing 1 to 2 pounds per week. You must burn 3500 Calories to lose 1 pound of fat. The goal is to increase energy expenditure by 350 to 500 Calories per day, 3 to 4 days per week. This is equivalent to 1050 to 2000 Calories expended per week. The remaining Calories can be reduced by decreasing daily caloric intake. Table 10 shows the energy cost of some common activities and how long it would take for a 150 lb. person to burn 350 Calories.

TABLE 10.   Caloric Cost of Activities

Activity	Calories Used per Hour	Time Needed to Use 350 Calories
Walking 2.5 mph	210	1 hr 40 min
Bicycling 5.5 mph	210	1 hr 40 min
Gardening	220	1 hr 36 min
Canoeing 2.5 mph	230	1 hr 31 min
Walking 3 mph	240	1 hr 27 min
Golf	250	1 hr 24 min
Walking 3.5 mph	270	1 hr 18 min
Swimming	300	1 hr 10 min
Walking 4 mph	300	1 hr 10 min
Softball	325	1 hr 4 min
Square dancing	350	1 hr
Tennis singles	420	50 min
Jogging 6 mph	600	35 min
Cross-country skiing	900	23 min
Running 8 mph	975	21 min
Running 10 mph	1200	18 min

Risk Factor Reduction

Coronary artery disease (CAD) is the major cause of death in the United States. It develops when fatty deposits build up on the inner walls of the blood vessels that supply the heart (coronary arteries), causing progressive narrowing. When the arteries become very narrow, the heart does not get adequate blood and the person begins to suffer angina (chest pain), or, if an artery is entirely obstructed, a heart attack may occur.

We now know that there are several risk factors that can increase your probability for developing CAD and thus the chances for having a heart attack. What are risk factors? Simply stated, risk factors are aspects of your lifestyle and habits or physical condition that influence the chances that you will develop coronary artery disease. Although not all risk factors can be eliminated, many can be reduced.

Considerable research sponsored by the National Institutes of Health, the American Heart Association, and other organizations has helped to identify these risks factors. One of the most important studies was conducted in Framingham, Massachusetts where 5000 adults were followed for over 25 years to determine which habits and conditions are linked to CAD. These risks factors are listed in Table 11.

The major risk factors are the ones that are particularly important to control, since each of these has been clearly linked to increased CAD. The higher the levels of these risk factors, the greater the risk. Furthermore, the risk factors multiply each other rather than add to each other. In other words, if you have one of the three major risk factors, your chances of developing CAD are doubled. As shown in Figure 6, if you have two, your chances are quadrupled, and if you have all three major risk factors, your chances are increased eight-fold!

Hypertension. Hypertension, or high blood pressure, afflicts 35 million people and is the most significant risk factor for both heart attack and

TABLE 11. Risk Factors for Developing Coronary Artery Disease

Major Risk Factors	Minor Risk Factors
1. Hypertension	1. Obesity
2. Elevated cholesterol	2. Diabetes
3. Cigarette smoking	3. Sedentary lifestyle
	4. Stress
	5. Family history of heart disease

(By permission of the American Heart Association, Inc.)

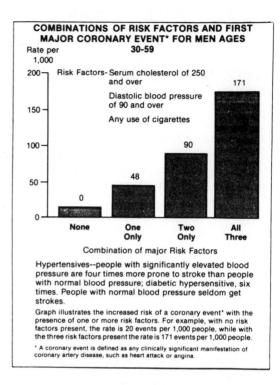

COMBINATIONS OF RISK FACTORS AND FIRST MAJOR CORONARY EVENT* FOR MEN AGES 30-59

Rate per 1,000

Risk Factors- Serum cholesterol of 250 and over

Diastolic blood pressure of 90 and over

Any use of cigarettes

Combination of major Risk Factors

Hypertensives--people with significantly elevated blood pressure are four times more prone to stroke than people with normal blood pressure; diabetic hypersensitive, six times. People with normal blood pressure seldom get strokes.

Graph illustrates the increased risk of a coronary event* with the presence of one or more risk factors. For example, with no risk factors present, the rate is 20 events per 1,000 people, while with the three risk factors present the rate is 171 events per 1,000 people.

* A coronary event is defined as any clinically significant manifestation of coronary artery disease, such as heart attack or angina.

Fig. 6 Coronary risk factors. By permission of the American Heart Association, Inc.

stroke. Every adult should have his or her blood pressure checked on a yearly basis to detect hypertension. Over 70% of individuals with hypertension have a mild form (diastolic blood pressure of 90–104). For these individuals weight loss, salt restriction, and sometimes stress reduction can help to lower blood pressure. Regular exercise has been shown to be an important component in sustained weight loss and therefore may play an important indirect role in blood pressure control.

Elevated Cholesterol. Elevated blood cholesterol is the second major risk factor for developing CAD. Cholesterol is a naturally occurring, waxy substance with a number of essential biological functions. We get cholesterol from two sources—our bodies manufacture it, and we get it from foods we eat. When there is too much cholesterol in the blood stream, it may be deposited on the inner walls of arteries, forming a fatty plaque.

Eggs, dairy products, and red meat are high in cholesterol content. The amount of cholesterol in your diet can be modified by limiting your intake of these foods. The American Heart Association recommends that no more than 30% of your Calories should be in fats, and half of those should be in unsaturated fats.

Cigarette Smoking. In 1979, the U.S. Surgeon General's report listed cigarette smoking as the Number 1 preventable cause of death in America. Cigarette smoking damages both the lungs and heart. Cigarette smokers are 30 times more likely to develop lung cancer than nonsmokers. If you smoke more than a pack of cigarettes a day, your chances of suffering a heart attack increase three-fold.

Smoking cessation results in a decrease in the risk of death from heart disease by approximately 50% after 1 year. Risk approaches that of a nonsmoker after 10 years. There are a number of smoking cessation programs available at local hospitals. The American Heart, Lung, and Cancer associations also provide information and programs for stopping smoking.

Other Risk Factors. The minor risk factors are also important but the linkages are less well established. Diabetes doubles the risk of CAD. Obesity or excess weight increases the likelihood of getting high blood pressure, high cholesterol, and diabetes. Being physically inactive also increases the risk of a heart attack. Compared to physically active people, inactive individuals have 1.5 to 2 times the risk of having a heart attack. The chance of dying suddenly is 3 times greater in inactive people.

Excessive stress also seems to predispose people to CAD as well as other chronic illnesses. A certain amount of stress may be necessary for some people to perform at their best. Excessive stress, however, can be a definite health hazard. It is essential for everyone to have periods of relaxation to combat stress. Stress-management programs are available at many hospitals.

A family history of heart disease means that you have had a blood relative below the age of 60 who has suffered a heart attack or stroke. Although you obviously cannot control your family history, you can pay extra close attention to controlling your risk factors if you have a family history of CAD or stroke.

Staying With It

The major health benefits of exercise are the result of a lifelong, consistent exercise program. This is termed *adherence* or *compliance*. Studies have shown that college or even Olympic athletes who stop exercising when their competitive careers are over revert to the same risk of developing heart disease as if they had never exercised at all.

Approximately 50% of those individuals who join an exercise program drop out within 6 weeks to 6 months. If you are just beginning a regular exercise program, the following considerations can help you develop a lifelong habit of exercise.

1. **Progress slowly.** If you have not exercised for a long time, you should progress slowly and not try to get back into shape in a couple of weeks. Start out with a brisk walk for 10 to 15 minutes and work up to higher-intensity and longer-duration exercise.
2. **Be regular.** Set aside certain times of the day to exercise. Put this time on your schedule so other activities will not conflict.
3. **Keep charts to record workouts.** These demonstrate progress and give positive feedback.
4. **Exercise with a friend or in groups.** Exercise may be more enjoyable with friends. Also, having to make commitments to friends can be a form of motivation and can help to ensure that you exercise on a regular schedule.
5. **Include variety.** Change exercise routes or routines or try alternative activities to enhance enjoyment and avoid boredom.
6. **Set short goals and provide rewards for yourself when you meet them.**
7. **Choose motivational equipment.** Computerized exercise equipment is now available, which may enhance enjoyment.

Summary

A program of total fitness should focus on both *health* and *exercise*. Aerobic conditioning, flexibility, strength training, proper nutrition, achieving desirable body weight, controlling blood pressure, avoiding cigarettes, and controlling stress are all important in a comprehensive program.

For Further Information

Books

The American Heart Association Cookbook. New York: David McKay Company, 1986.
Anderson, Robert, *Stretching*. Bolinas, CA: Shelter Publications, Inc., 1980.
Cooper, Kenneth, *Aerobics Program for Total Well-Being*. New York: Bantam Books, 1983.

Getchall, Bud, *Physical Fitness, A Way of Life.* New York: John Wiley & Sons, 1976.

Kashiwa A, Rippe JM: Fitness Walking for Women. New York: Putnam Publishing Co., 1987.

Katch, Frank I. and William D. McArdle, *Nutrition, Weight Control & Exercise.* Philadelphia: Lea & Febiger, 1983.

Rippe, James M. and William Southmayd, *The Sports Performance Factors.* New York: Putnam Publishing Co., 1986.

Sweetgall, Robert, James M. Rippe, and Frank Katch, *Fitness Walking.* New York: Putnam Publishing Co., 1985.

Pamphlets

The Rockport Fitness Walking Test. Marlboro, MA: Rockport Walking Institute, 1987.

Staying With It. Life Fitness, President's Council on Physical Fitness, 1987.

Walking. Marlboro, MA: Rockport Walking Institute, 1987.

Ward, Ann and James M. Rippe, *Walking for Health and Fitness.* Philadelphia: J. B. Lippincott Co., 1988.

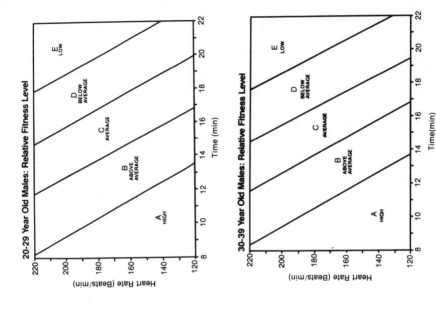

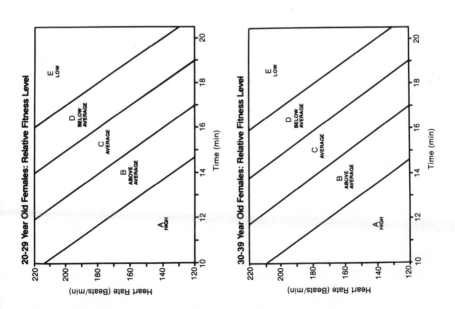

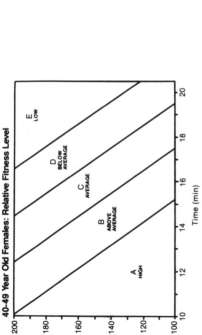

40-49 Year Old Females: Relative Fitness Level

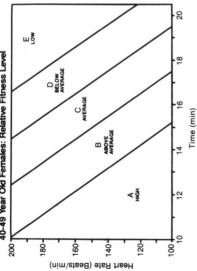

50-59 Year Old Females: Relative Fitness Level

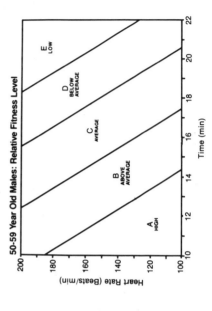

40-49 Year Old Males: Relative Fitness Level

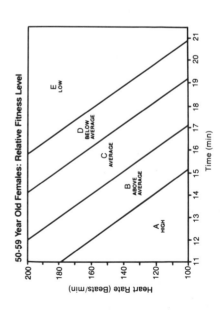

50-59 Year Old Males: Relative Fitness Level

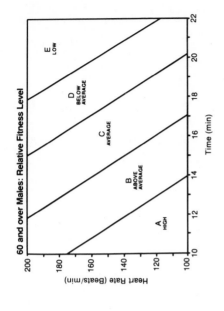

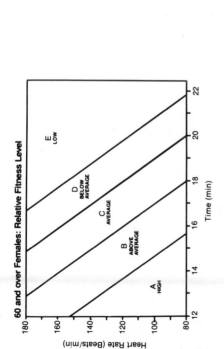